ENDURING HOPE

Enduring Hope

Supporting a Loved One with Chronic Suicidal Thoughts

CHRISTOPHER BENTLEY

Advise the Heart

CONTENTS

First Printing, 2024

ISBN/SKU979-8-8692-7306-2
EISBN979-8-8692-7307-9

Disclaimer: This book is intended to provide guidance and support for individuals helping a loved one through a mental health crisis. It is not a substitute for professional medical advice, diagnosis, or treatment. Readers are encouraged to seek the assistance of qualified mental health professionals for personalized recommendations and interventions.

In cases where there is an immediate threat to the safety or well-being of the individual or others, readers are strongly advised to contact local emergency services or a crisis hotline for immediate assistance. The author and publisher do not assume any responsibility for actions taken based on the information provided in this book. Readers should use their judgment and consult with appropriate professionals when making decisions related to mental health crises.

An Important Note

For concerned loved ones whose family members, friends, partners, children, coworkers, spouses, siblings, or caregivers are struggling with chronic suicidal thoughts, it can be an incredibly challenging and heartbreaking experience. It's important to remember that you are not alone in this journey, and there is hope for your loved one's recovery.

One of the most important things you can do for someone with chronic suicidal thoughts is to listen and show your support without judgment. Let them know that you are there for them, that you care about them, and that you want to help them through this difficult time. Encourage them to seek professional help, whether that means therapy, medication, or other forms of treatment. Be patient with them as they navigate their journey towards healing.

It's also crucial to educate yourself about suicide and mental health issues. Understanding the warning signs of suicidal behavior, knowing how to talk to your loved one about their thoughts and feelings, and being aware of available resources can make a significant difference in their recovery process.

Remember to take care of yourself as well. Supporting someone with chronic suicidal thoughts can take a toll on your own mental and emotional well-being. Reach out to a therapist, counselor, support group, or trusted friend for help and guidance. Practice self-care activities such as exercise, meditation, and spending time with loved ones to recharge and rejuvenate.

Above all, hold onto hope. Recovery is possible, and with your unwavering love and support, your loved one can find the strength to overcome their struggles and build a brighter future. Together, you can endure this challenging journey and emerge stronger and more resilient than ever before.

| 1 |

Understanding Suicidal Thoughts

Recognizing the Signs of Suicidal Ideation

As a concerned loved one, it is crucial to be able to recognize the signs of suicidal ideation in your family member, friend, partner, child, co-worker, spouse, sibling, or loved one. By being aware of these signs, you can intervene and provide the necessary support and resources to help them through this difficult time.

One of the most common signs of suicidal ideation is talking about wanting to die or feeling hopeless and trapped. Your loved one may also express feelings of worthlessness or guilt, and may withdraw from social activities or isolate themselves from others. Changes in behavior, such as increased use of drugs or alcohol, reckless behavior, or giving away possessions, can also be warning signs of suicidal ideation.

It is important to take any mention of suicide seriously and not dismiss it as attention-seeking behavior. If you notice any of these signs in your loved one, it is crucial to have an open and honest conversation with them about how they are feeling. Encourage them to seek help from a mental health professional and offer your support in finding resources and treatment options.

Remember, suicidal ideation is a serious mental health issue that requires professional intervention. By recognizing the signs of suicidal ideation and offering your loved one support and guidance, you can help them navigate through this challenging time and provide them with the hope and encouragement they need to heal and recover.

Together, we can support our loved ones through their struggles and help them find enduring hope.

Understanding the Root Causes of Suicidal Thoughts

In order to effectively support a loved one dealing with chronic suicidal thoughts, it is crucial to understand the root causes behind these thoughts. While every individual's experience is unique, there are common factors that can contribute to suicidal ideation.

One of the primary factors is mental illness, such as depression, anxiety, bipolar disorder, or schizophrenia. These conditions can distort a person's perception of reality and make it difficult for them to see a way out of their pain. It is important to recognize the signs of mental illness and seek professional help for your loved one.

Traumatic experiences, such as abuse, bullying, or the loss of a loved one, can also trigger suicidal thoughts. These experiences can leave lasting emotional scars and make it challenging for individuals to cope with their feelings. Providing a safe and supportive environment for your loved one to process their trauma is essential in helping them heal.

Feelings of hopelessness, helplessness, and worthlessness can also contribute to suicidal ideation. Your loved one may feel like they are a burden to others or that their life has no purpose. It is important to validate their feelings and remind them of their inherent worth and value as a person.

Substance abuse, chronic pain, and financial struggles are other common factors that can exacerbate suicidal thoughts. These issues can compound a person's existing struggles and make it even harder for them to see a way forward. It is important to address these underlying issues and provide your loved one with the necessary support and resources to overcome them.

By understanding the root causes of your loved one's suicidal thoughts, you can better support them on their journey towards healing and recovery. Remember, you are not alone in this journey, and there are resources and professionals available to help you navigate this challenging time.

Common Myths and Misconceptions About Suicide

In our society, there are many myths and misconceptions surrounding the topic of suicide. These misconceptions can often prevent people from seeking help or offering support to loved ones who are struggling with suicidal thoughts. As concerned loved ones, it is crucial to educate ourselves on the truth behind these myths in order to better support those in need.

One common myth about suicide is that talking about it will only make things worse. This is not true. In fact, talking openly and honestly about suicidal thoughts can be incredibly beneficial for individuals who are struggling. It allows them to feel heard, understood, and supported, which can reduce feelings of isolation and hopelessness.

Another myth is that people who talk about suicide are just seeking attention. This is a dangerous misconception that can lead to dismissive attitudes towards those in need. It is important to take all mentions of suicide seriously and to offer help and support to anyone who may be struggling.

Many people also believe that once someone has made a suicide attempt, they will not try again. This is simply not the case. Suicide is often a result of deep emotional pain and distress, and individuals who have attempted suicide may still be at risk. It is crucial to continue offering support and monitoring their well-being.

By debunking these common myths and misconceptions about suicide, concerned loved ones can better understand how to support those struggling with suicidal thoughts. It is important to approach the topic with empathy, compassion, and a willingness to listen. Together, we can help break the stigma surrounding suicide and provide the necessary support for those in need.

| 2 |

Helping a Loved One Through Suicidal Thoughts

Opening the Lines of Communication

One of the most important steps in supporting a loved one with chronic suicidal thoughts is to open the lines of communication. It can be challenging to broach the topic of suicide, but avoiding the conversation will not make the thoughts or feelings go away. By initiating an open and honest dialogue, you can create a safe space for your loved one to express their thoughts and emotions.

When starting a conversation about suicide, it is important to approach the topic with empathy and compassion. Let your loved one know that you are there for them and that you want to listen without judgment. Encourage them to share their feelings and thoughts, and assure them that they are not alone in their struggles.

As you talk with your loved one, it is important to actively listen to what they are saying. Validate their feelings and let them know that you hear them. Avoid offering unsolicited advice or trying to "fix" their problems, as this can make them feel invalidated. Instead, focus on being a supportive presence and offering your unconditional love and care.

In addition to listening, it is important to ask direct questions about suicidal thoughts or intentions. While this may feel uncomfortable, it is crucial to assess the level of risk and determine the appropriate course of action. If you believe that your loved one is in immediate danger, do not hesitate to seek help from a mental health professional or emergency services.

By opening the lines of communication with

your loved one, you can create a foundation of trust and support that is essential for their healing journey. Remember, you are not alone in this process, and there are resources available to help you navigate the complexities of supporting a loved one with chronic suicidal thoughts.

Providing Emotional Support and Understanding

As a concerned loved one of someone struggling with chronic suicidal thoughts, it is crucial to provide emotional support and understanding to help them navigate their difficult journey. It is important to remember that suicidal thoughts are a symptom of deep emotional pain and should not be dismissed or trivialized. Your loved one needs to feel heard, valued, and supported during this challenging time.

One of the most important things you can do is to actively listen to your loved one without judgment. Let them know that you are there for them, that you care about them, and that you want to help them through this difficult time. Encourage them to open up about their thoughts and feelings, and validate their emotions without trying to fix or minimize them.

Offering empathy and understanding can go a long way in helping your loved one feel supported and less alone in their struggles. Let them know that it is okay to feel the way they do, and that you are there to support them through their darkest moments. Reassure them that they are not a burden and that their feelings are valid.

Additionally, educate yourself about mental health and suicide prevention resources so that you can provide your loved one with the support and guidance they need. Encourage them to seek professional help and accompany them to therapy sessions or support groups if needed.

Above all, remember that providing emotional support and understanding to your loved one is a continuous process. Be patient, kind, and compassionate, and let them know that you are there for them every step of the way. Your unwavering support can make a world of difference in their journey towards healing and recovery.

Encouraging Professional Help and Treatment Options

When supporting a loved one with chronic suicidal thoughts, it is crucial to encourage them to seek professional help and explore treatment options. As concerned loved ones, it can be overwhelming to witness someone we care about struggling with such intense and potentially life-threatening emotions. However, it is important to remember that we are not equipped to provide the level of support and intervention that a trained mental health professional can offer.

One of the first steps in encouraging professional help is to have an open and honest conversation with your loved one about their suicidal thoughts. Express your concerns in a non-judgmental and empathetic manner, and let them know that you are there to support them in finding the help they need. Encourage them to speak with a therapist, counselor, or psychiatrist who specializes in treating individuals with suicidal ideation.

Additionally, it may be helpful to research and provide information on different treatment options available, such as therapy, medication, support groups, and hospitalization if necessary. Be proactive in helping your loved one schedule appointments and follow through with treatment recommendations.

It is also important to take care of yourself as a concerned loved one. Supporting someone with chronic suicidal thoughts can be emotionally draining, so be sure to prioritize your own well-being and seek support from friends, family, or a therapist if needed.

Remember, professional help and treatment options are essential in helping your loved one navigate their suicidal thoughts and find hope for the future. By encouraging them to seek help, you are showing them that they are not alone in their struggles and that there is a path towards healing and recovery.

| 3 |

Supporting Family Members with Suicidal Thoughts

Navigating Family Dynamics and Communication

When a loved one is struggling with chronic suicidal thoughts, it can be incredibly challenging to navigate the complex dynamics of family relationships. Communication is key in these situations, but it can often be fraught with tension, misunderstandings, and emotional turmoil. As a concerned loved one, it is important to approach these delicate conversations with empathy, understanding, and patience.

One of the first steps in navigating family dynamics and communication is to create a safe and non-judgmental space for your loved one to express their feelings. Let them know that you are there to listen, support, and help them through this difficult time. Encourage open and honest communication, but also respect their boundaries and privacy.

It is also important to educate yourself about mental health and suicide prevention. Understanding the warning signs, risk factors, and available resources can help you provide the best possible support for your loved one. Consider attending therapy or support groups together to learn effective communication strategies and coping mechanisms.

When communicating with family members about your loved one's suicidal thoughts, it is important to approach the conversation with sensitivity and empathy. Avoid placing blame or judgment, and instead focus on finding solutions and offering support. Encourage open dialogue, active listening, and validation of each other's feelings.

Remember that navigating family dynamics and communication is an ongoing process that requires patience, understanding, and compassion. By actively working together to support your loved one, you can create a strong foundation of love and understanding that will help them through their struggles with chronic suicidal thoughts.

Creating a Safe and Supportive Environment at Home

Creating a safe and supportive environment at home is crucial when supporting a loved one with chronic suicidal thoughts. As concerned loved ones, it is important to understand the impact of the home environment on an individual's mental health and well-being. By taking proactive steps to create a safe and supportive space, you can help your loved one feel more secure and cared for.

One of the first steps in creating a safe environment is to remove any potential hazards or triggers that may contribute to your loved one's suicidal thoughts. This could include safely storing medications, firearms, or other potentially harmful items. It is also important to create a calm and peaceful atmosphere at home, free from unnecessary stress or conflict.

In addition to physical safety, it is important to provide emotional support to your loved one. Listen to their thoughts and feelings without judgment, and validate their experiences. Encourage open communication and let them know that they are not alone in their struggles. Offer reassurance and comfort, and remind them of your love and support.

Creating a routine and structure at home can also help your loved one feel more stable and secure. Establishing regular mealtimes, sleep schedules, and activities can provide a sense of predictability and control. Encourage healthy habits such as exercise, relaxation techniques, and self-care activities.

Finally, it is important to seek professional help and support for your loved one. Connect them with a therapist, counselor, or support group who can provide specialized care and resources. Remember that you are not alone in this journey, and there are many resources available to help you support your loved one through their struggles with chronic suicidal thoughts.

Building a Strong Support System Within the Family

One of the most important things you can do for a loved one struggling with chronic suicidal thoughts is to build a strong support system within the family. This support system can provide the foundation for your loved one's recovery and help them feel less isolated in their struggles.

First and foremost, it's crucial to communicate openly and honestly with your loved one about their feelings and thoughts. Encourage them to share their emotions and fears without judgment, and let them know that you are there to listen and support them unconditionally.

In addition to open communication, it's essential to educate yourself about suicide and mental health issues. Understanding the warning signs and risk factors of suicide can help you better support your loved one and know when to seek professional help.

Creating a safe and supportive environment within the family is also key. Encourage your loved one to engage in self-care activities, such as exercise, meditation, or spending time with loved ones. Make sure they have access to mental health resources and support groups, and encourage them to seek help when needed.

Finally, remember to take care of yourself as well. Supporting a loved one with chronic suicidal thoughts can be emotionally draining, so it's important to prioritize your own mental health and well-being. Seek support from friends, family, or a therapist, and don't be afraid to ask for help when you need it.

By building a strong support system within the family, you can help your loved one feel less alone in their struggles and provide them with the love and encouragement they need to overcome their suicidal thoughts. Remember, you are not alone in this journey, and there is hope for a brighter future ahead.

| 4 |

Assisting Friends Coping with Suicidal Ideation

Approaching the Topic of Suicide with a Friend

Approaching the topic of suicide with a friend can be a daunting and sensitive task, but it is crucial in providing support and potentially saving a life. As a concerned loved one, it is important to approach the conversation with empathy, understanding, and an open mind.

First and foremost, create a safe and comfortable space for your friend to talk openly about their feelings. Let them know that you are there to listen without judgment and that you care about their well-being. Express your concern for their safety and reassure them that their thoughts and feelings are valid.

It is important to ask direct questions about suicide, such as if they have a plan or intention to harm themselves. Encourage them to seek professional help and offer to help them find resources, such as a therapist or hotline. Do not try to handle the situation alone, as it is crucial to involve trained professionals in supporting your friend.

Be prepared for a range of emotions from your friend, including anger, sadness, and fear. Stay calm and patient, and do not take any negative reactions personally. Remember that your friend is struggling with intense emotions and may not be thinking clearly.

Lastly, follow up with your friend regularly and continue to offer your support. Check in on their well-being and encourage them to seek help if needed. Remind them that they are not alone in their struggles and that there is hope for healing and recovery.

Approaching the topic of suicide with a friend can be challenging, but your willingness to listen and support them can make a significant difference in their journey towards healing. Remember to prioritize their safety and well-being above all else.

Being a Source of Comfort and Understanding

Being a source of comfort and understanding for a loved one struggling with chronic suicidal thoughts is incredibly important. When someone is in such a dark place, they may feel isolated and alone. As a concerned loved one, your role is to provide a safe space for them to open up and share their feelings without judgment.

One of the most crucial ways to be supportive is to actively listen to what your loved one is going through. Let them know that you are there for them and that you care about their well-being.

Avoid offering unsolicited advice or trying to "fix" their problems. Sometimes, all they need is someone to listen and validate their feelings.

It's also essential to educate yourself about suicide and mental health. Understanding the warning signs and risk factors associated with suicidal thoughts can help you better support your loved one. Encourage them to seek professional help and offer to accompany them to therapy or doctor's appointments.

In addition to being a listening ear, try to engage in activities that bring joy and comfort to your loved one. Whether it's going for a walk, watching a movie together, or simply spending quality time, these small gestures can make a big difference in their mental well-being.

Remember to take care of yourself as well while supporting your loved one. It's okay to set boundaries and seek support from friends, family, or a therapist if you feel overwhelmed. By being a source of comfort and understanding, you can help your loved one navigate their struggles and find hope for the future.

Encouraging Professional Help and Resources for Support

When supporting a loved one with chronic suicidal thoughts, it is crucial to recognize the importance of seeking professional help and utilizing available resources for support. As concerned loved ones, it can be overwhelming and daunting to navigate the complexities of dealing with someone who is struggling with suicidal ideation. However, it is essential to remember that you do not have to go through this alone.

One of the most effective ways to help your loved one is by encouraging them to seek professional help. This may include therapy, counseling, or psychiatric treatment. Professional mental health professionals are trained to provide the necessary support and guidance to individuals dealing with suicidal thoughts. They can offer a safe space for your loved one to express their feelings and work through their struggles in a healthy and constructive manner.

Additionally, as a concerned loved one, it is important to educate yourself on the available resources and support systems in your community. This may include hotlines, support groups, crisis intervention services, and online resources. By being informed about these resources, you can better assist your loved one in finding the help they need.

Remember, supporting a loved one with chronic suicidal thoughts can be emotionally draining and challenging. It is crucial to take care of yourself as well and seek support from friends, family, or a therapist. By prioritizing your own well-being, you can better support your loved one in their journey towards healing and recovery.

In conclusion, encouraging professional help and utilizing available resources for support is essential when helping a loved one with chronic suicidal thoughts. By working together with mental health professionals and accessing the necessary resources, you can provide the best possible support for your loved one during this difficult time.

| 5 |

Providing Guidance for Parents of a Child with Suicidal Thoughts

Recognizing the Signs of Suicide Risk in Children

As concerned loved ones, it is crucial to be aware of the signs that may indicate a child is at risk for suicide. While it can be difficult to imagine a child experiencing such intense emotions, it is important to take any signs seriously and seek help immediately.

One of the most common signs of suicide risk

in children is a sudden change in behavior. This could include withdrawing from activities they once enjoyed, isolating themselves from friends and family, or displaying extreme mood swings. Children who talk about feeling hopeless, worthless, or like a burden to others may also be at risk for suicide.

Physical symptoms such as changes in appetite, sleep patterns, or energy levels can also be red flags. Keep an eye out for signs of self-harm, such as unexplained cuts or bruises, as well.

It is important to remember that children may not always express their emotions verbally. Pay attention to any changes in their artwork, writing, or social media posts, as these can provide important insights into their mental state.

If you suspect a child is at risk for suicide, it is crucial to take action immediately. Talk to them openly and honestly about your concerns, and offer your support and understanding. Encourage them to seek professional help, such as therapy or counseling, and make sure they know they are not alone in their struggles.

By recognizing the signs of suicide risk in children and taking proactive steps to address them, you can help support your loved one through their darkest moments and guide them towards a path of healing and hope.

Communicating with Children About Mental Health and Suicide

Communicating with children about mental health and suicide is a delicate and crucial task for concerned loved ones. It is important to approach this topic with sensitivity, honesty, and empathy in order to provide the necessary support and resources for the child in need.

When discussing mental health and suicide with children, it is important to use age-appropriate language and concepts. Avoid using confusing or frightening terminology, and instead focus on explaining emotions and thoughts in a simple and clear manner. Encourage open and honest communication, and let the child know that it is safe to talk about their feelings without judgment.

Listen actively to the child's concerns and validate their emotions. Let them know that it is okay to feel sad, scared, or overwhelmed, and reassure them that they are not alone in their struggles. Provide them with resources such as hotlines, support groups, or therapy options, and encourage them to reach out for help when needed.

It is also important to create a safe and supportive environment for the child at home and in their community. Help them establish healthy coping mechanisms, such as journaling, art therapy, or mindfulness exercises, and encourage them to engage in activities that bring them joy and relaxation.

Above all, remind the child that they are loved and valued, and that their mental health is just as important as their physical well-being. By communicating openly and compassionately about mental health and suicide, concerned loved ones can provide the necessary support for children struggling with these issues.

Seeking Professional Help for Child Suicidal Thoughts

Seeking professional help for a child experiencing suicidal thoughts is crucial in ensuring their safety and well-being. As concerned loved ones, it is important to recognize the signs and symptoms of suicidal ideation in children and take immediate action to get them the help they need.

When a child expresses thoughts of suicide or exhibits concerning behaviors such as withdrawing from activities they once enjoyed, giving away prized possessions, or talking about feeling hopeless, it is essential to seek help from a mental health professional. This could be a therapist, counselor, psychologist, or psychiatrist who specializes in working with children and adolescents.

Professional help can provide a child with the necessary support, therapy, and interventions to address the underlying issues contributing to their suicidal thoughts. Therapists can help children develop coping strategies, improve their emotional regulation skills, and build resilience to better navigate challenging situations.

In addition to therapy, medication may also be recommended by a psychiatrist to help manage any underlying mental health conditions such as depression or anxiety that may be contributing to the child's suicidal thoughts.

As concerned loved ones, it is important to offer your support and encouragement to the child throughout their treatment journey. Be patient, understanding, and non-judgmental as they navigate their feelings and experiences. Remember that seeking professional help is a positive step towards healing and recovery for the child.

By seeking professional help for a child experiencing suicidal thoughts, you are taking a proactive approach to ensuring their safety and providing them with the necessary support to overcome their struggles. Remember, you are not alone in this journey, and there are resources and professionals available to help you and your child through this difficult time.

| 6 |

Supporting a Partner Through Suicidal Tendencies

Strengthening the Bond and Connection with Your Partner

When supporting a partner through chronic suicidal thoughts, it is crucial to focus on strengthening the bond and connection between the two of you. Building a strong foundation of trust, communication, and understanding can make a significant difference in your loved one's recovery journey. Here are some tips for fostering a stronger bond with your partner:

1. Open and honest communication: En-

courage your partner to express their thoughts and feelings openly and honestly. Create a safe space where they feel comfortable sharing their struggles without fear of judgment.

2. Active listening: Practice active listening by giving your partner your full attention when they are speaking. Show empathy and understanding by reflecting back what they are saying and validating their emotions.
3. Quality time together: Make an effort to spend quality time together doing activities that you both enjoy. This can help strengthen your connection and provide a welcome distraction from negative thoughts.
4. Support their treatment plan: Encourage your partner to seek professional help and support them in their treatment journey. Attend therapy sessions together if appropriate and help them stay on track with medications and appointments.
5. Show love and affection: Small gestures of love and affection can go a long way in showing your partner that you care. Physical

touch, words of affirmation, and acts of kindness can all help strengthen your bond.

By focusing on building a strong and supportive relationship with your partner, you can help them feel loved, valued, and understood as they navigate their struggles with chronic suicidal thoughts. Remember, you are not alone in this journey, and there are resources available to support both you and your loved one.

Offering Unconditional Love and Support

When a loved one is struggling with chronic suicidal thoughts, it can be an incredibly challenging and heartbreaking experience. As a concerned loved one, it is natural to want to do everything in your power to help and support them through this difficult time. One of the most important things you can offer them is your unconditional love and support.

It is crucial to remember that your loved one is going through a deep and painful emotional struggle, and they may feel overwhelmed and alone. By offering them your unwavering love and support, you can help them feel validated, understood, and cared for.

One way to demonstrate your unconditional love and support is by actively listening to your loved one without judgment. Allow them to express their thoughts and feelings openly and honestly, and let them know that you are there for them no matter what. Avoid offering unsolicited advice or trying to "fix" their problems, as this can make them feel invalidated and misunderstood.

Additionally, make sure to check in on your loved one regularly and remind them that you are there for them whenever they need you. Offer to spend time with them, engage in activities they enjoy, and provide a comforting presence during times of distress.

Above all, remind your loved one that they are not alone in their struggles and that you are committed to supporting them through thick and thin. Your unconditional love and support can make a world of difference in their recovery journey and help them feel less isolated and hopeless.

Remember, offering unconditional love and support to a loved one with chronic suicidal thoughts is a powerful way to show them that they are valued, cared for, and not alone in their struggles. Your unwavering presence can provide them with the strength and reassurance they need to keep fighting for a brighter tomorrow.

Helping Your Partner Seek Professional Help and Treatment

If you suspect that your partner is struggling with chronic suicidal thoughts, it is crucial to encourage them to seek professional help and treatment. It can be a daunting task to broach this subject, but it is essential for their well-being and safety. Here are some steps you can take to support your partner in seeking the help they need:

1. Open a dialogue: Approach your partner with empathy and understanding. Let them

know that you are concerned about their well-being and that you are there to support them. Encourage them to share their feelings and thoughts with you.

2. Research treatment options: Take the time to research different treatment options available for individuals struggling with suicidal thoughts. This could include therapy, medication, support groups, or inpatient treatment. Present these options to your partner in a non-judgmental way.
3. Offer to accompany them: Going to therapy or seeking treatment can be a scary and overwhelming experience. Offer to accompany your partner to their appointments for moral support. Let them know that they are not alone in this journey.
4. Be patient and understanding: Recovery from chronic suicidal thoughts takes time and effort. Be patient with your partner and offer them unconditional love and support throughout the process. Encourage them to stick with their treatment plan, even when it gets tough.
5. Provide resources: Connect your partner

with resources and hotlines that can offer immediate support in times of crisis. Make sure they have access to emergency services if needed.

Remember, it is okay to seek help for yourself as well. Taking care of your own mental health is essential in supporting your partner through this difficult time. By working together and seeking professional help, you can help your partner find hope and healing.

| 7 |

Helping a Spouse Through Suicidal Struggles

Understanding the Impact of Suicide on a Marriage

When a partner in a marriage is struggling with chronic suicidal thoughts, it can have a profound impact on the relationship as a whole. The constant fear and worry about their safety can put a significant strain on the marriage, leading to feelings of helplessness, frustration, and sadness for both individuals involved.

For the spouse of someone with suicidal tendencies, it can be overwhelming to constantly be on high alert and trying to prevent any harm from coming to their loved one. This can lead to feelings of anxiety, stress, and even resentment towards their partner for putting them in this position.

Communication in a marriage where one partner is dealing with suicidal thoughts is crucial. It is important for both individuals to be open and honest about their feelings and fears, and to create a safe space for each other to express themselves without judgment. Seeking couples therapy or counseling can also be beneficial in navigating these difficult conversations and finding ways to support each other through this challenging time.

It is also important for the spouse to take care of their own mental health during this time. It is not selfish to prioritize self-care and seek support for themselves, as they cannot effectively support their partner if they are not taking care of themselves first.

By understanding the impact of suicide on a marriage and actively working together to navigate these challenges, couples can strengthen their bond and support each other through even the most difficult times. Remember, you are not alone in this journey, and there are resources and support available to help you through.

Navigating Intense Emotions and Challenges Together

Navigating intense emotions and challenges together when supporting a loved one with chronic suicidal thoughts can be overwhelming and exhausting. It is crucial for concerned loved ones to prioritize self-care and seek support from others who understand the unique difficulties they are facing.

One of the most important things to remember is to listen without judgment. Your loved one may be experiencing intense emotions and may not always express themselves in a way that is easy to understand. It is important to provide a safe space for them to talk about their feelings and thoughts without fear of being criticized or dismissed.

Additionally, it is important to educate yourself

about the warning signs of suicidal ideation and how to help your loved one access the support they need. This may involve connecting them with mental health professionals, crisis hotlines, or support groups where they can find understanding and compassionate individuals who can help them navigate their struggles.

As a concerned loved one, it is also important to set boundaries and take care of your own mental health. It is easy to become consumed by your loved one's struggles, but it is important to remember that you cannot pour from an empty cup. Take time to engage in self-care activities, seek therapy for yourself if needed, and lean on your own support system for help.

Remember, you are not alone in this journey. There are resources available to help you navigate the intense emotions and challenges that come with supporting a loved one with chronic suicidal thoughts. By taking care of yourself and seeking support when needed, you can better support your loved one through their struggles and help them find hope and healing.

Moving Forward and Rebuilding Trust After a Suicide Crisis

After a loved one has experienced a suicide crisis, it can be difficult to know how to move forward and rebuild trust. The aftermath of a suicide attempt or chronic suicidal thoughts can leave everyone involved feeling overwhelmed, confused, and unsure of how to proceed. However, it is possible to navigate this challenging time with patience, understanding, and support.

One of the most important things to remember as a concerned loved one is to be patient with both yourself and your loved one. It is normal to feel a range of emotions after a suicide crisis, including anger, guilt, sadness, and confusion. Allow yourself to experience these feelings without judgment and seek support from a therapist or support group if needed.

In order to rebuild trust with your loved one, it is essential to continue to communicate openly and honestly. Let them know that you are there for them, no matter what, and that you are committed to supporting them through their struggles. Be willing to listen without judgment and offer your unconditional love and support.

It is also important to establish healthy boundaries in your relationship with your loved one. While it is natural to want to protect them and prevent future crises, it is not your responsibility to fix their problems or monitor their every move. Encourage them to seek professional help and support them in their journey towards healing and recovery.

By taking these steps and approaching the situation with compassion and understanding, you can begin to rebuild trust with your loved one and move forward together towards a brighter future. Remember, you are not alone in this journey, and there are resources and support available to help you navigate this challenging time.

| 8 |

Assisting Siblings with Suicidal Ideation

Building a Supportive Relationship with Your Sibling

When it comes to supporting a sibling who is struggling with chronic suicidal thoughts, building a strong and supportive relationship is crucial. As a concerned loved one, your sibling may turn to you for support, guidance, and understanding during their darkest moments. Here are some tips on how to cultivate a supportive relationship with your sibling:

1. Listen without judgment: One of the most important things you can do for your sibling is to listen to them without passing judgment. Allow them to express their feelings and thoughts without fear of criticism or rejection. Let them know that you are there to support them unconditionally.
2. Validate their feelings: It is essential to validate your sibling's feelings and emotions, even if you may not fully understand them. Let them know that it is okay to feel the way they do and that their feelings are valid.
3. Offer practical support: In addition to emotional support, offer practical help to your sibling. This could include helping them find a therapist, accompanying them to appointments, or assisting them with day-to-day tasks when they are struggling.
4. Educate yourself: Take the time to educate yourself about suicidal thoughts and behaviors. Understanding the warning signs and risk factors can help you better support your sibling and know when to seek professional help.
5. Encourage open communication: En-

courage your sibling to communicate openly with you about their thoughts and feelings. Let them know that they can come to you at any time, and that you are there to listen and support them.

By building a supportive relationship with your sibling, you can provide them with the love, understanding, and guidance they need to navigate their struggles with chronic suicidal thoughts. Remember, you are not alone in this journey, and there are resources available to help you support your sibling through their darkest moments.

Communicating Openly and Honestly About Suicidal Thoughts

Communicating openly and honestly about suicidal thoughts is crucial when supporting a loved one who is struggling. It can be a difficult and uncomfortable topic to broach, but it is essential for both their safety and your peace of mind. Here are some tips for having these difficult conversations with your loved one:

1. Create a safe and comfortable space for the conversation. Choose a time when you both are calm and can talk without interruptions. Let your loved one know that you are there to listen and support them.
2. Be direct and non-judgmental. Ask your loved one if they have been having thoughts of suicide and allow them to express their feelings without fear of being judged. Let them know that you care about them and want to help.
3. Listen actively and validate their feelings. Let your loved one know that it is okay to feel overwhelmed and that you are there to support them through their struggles. Avoid trying to minimize their feelings or offer quick solutions.
4. Encourage your loved one to seek professional help. Let them know that there are resources available to help them cope with their suicidal thoughts, such as therapy, support groups, and hotlines. Offer to help

them find a therapist or accompany them to appointments.

5. Follow up regularly. Check in with your loved one regularly to see how they are doing and to offer your support. Let them know that you are there for them no matter what and that they are not alone in their struggles.

Remember, talking about suicide does not increase the risk of someone acting on their thoughts. In fact, open and honest communication can help reduce the stigma surrounding mental health issues and encourage your loved one to seek help. By being a supportive and understanding presence in their life, you can help them navigate their struggles and find hope for the future.

Seeking Professional Help and Resources for Sibling Support

When a sibling is struggling with chronic suicidal thoughts, it can be overwhelming and heartbreaking for their loved ones. As a concerned sibling, it is important to seek professional help and resources to support your sibling through this difficult time.

One of the first steps you can take is to encourage your sibling to seek help from a mental health professional. This could be a therapist, counselor, psychiatrist, or psychologist who specializes in working with individuals who have suicidal thoughts. They can provide your sibling with the necessary support, guidance, and treatment to help them cope with their suicidal ideation.

Additionally, as a concerned loved one, you can also seek support for yourself. It is essential to take care of your own mental and emotional well-being during this challenging time. Consider reaching out to a therapist or support group for siblings of individuals with suicidal thoughts. Talking to others who are going through similar experiences can provide you with the understanding and comfort you need.

In addition to professional help, there are also resources available for siblings supporting a loved one with chronic suicidal thoughts. Organizations such as the National Alliance on Mental Illness (NAMI) and the American Foundation for Suicide Prevention offer valuable information, support groups, and resources for individuals and families affected by suicide.

Remember, you are not alone in this journey. By seeking professional help and resources, you can better support your sibling and navigate through this difficult time together. Your love, understanding, and commitment can make a significant difference in your sibling's recovery and healing process.

| 9 |

Providing Resources for Caregivers of Individuals with Suicidal Thoughts

Self-Care Tips and Strategies for Caregivers

Taking care of a loved one who is struggling with chronic suicidal thoughts can be incredibly challenging and emotionally draining. As a caregiver, it is important to prioritize your own well-being so that you can continue to provide support to your loved one. Here are some self-care tips and strategies for caregivers:

1. Seek support: It's essential to have a strong support system in place when caring for someone with chronic suicidal thoughts. Reach out to friends, family members, support groups, or a therapist to talk about your feelings and experiences.
2. Set boundaries: It's okay to set boundaries with your loved one to protect your own mental and emotional health. Make sure to communicate your needs and limitations clearly and assertively.
3. Take breaks: Caring for someone with chronic suicidal thoughts can be overwhelming. Make sure to take breaks when you need them and engage in activities that bring you joy and relaxation.
4. Practice self-care: Make time for self-care activities that help you recharge and de-stress. This could include exercise, meditation, reading, or spending time in nature.
5. Educate yourself: Knowledge is power, so take the time to educate yourself about suicide, mental health, and available resources. The more you know, the better equipped you will be to support your loved one.

Remember, you cannot pour from an empty cup. Taking care of yourself is not selfish – it is necessary in order to be able to effectively care for your loved one. By prioritizing your own well-being, you will be better able to provide the support and guidance your loved one needs during this difficult time.

Connecting with Support Groups and Mental Health Professionals

Connecting with support groups and mental health professionals can be a crucial step in helping your loved one navigate their chronic suicidal thoughts. These resources can provide valuable support, guidance, and tools for both your loved one and yourself as you navigate this challenging journey together.

Support groups specifically geared towards individuals struggling with suicidal thoughts can offer a sense of community and understanding that is often difficult to find elsewhere. These groups provide a safe space for individuals to share their experiences, fears, and challenges, and can offer valuable insights and coping strategies from others who have been in similar situations.

Mental health professionals, such as therapists, counselors, and psychiatrists, can also play a vital role in supporting your loved one. They are trained to help individuals work through their thoughts and emotions, develop healthy coping mechanisms, and identify and address underlying issues that may be contributing to their suicidal thoughts. Additionally, mental health professionals can provide valuable resources and referrals for additional support services, such as medication management or intensive therapy programs.

As a concerned loved one, it is important to remember that you do not have to navigate this journey alone. By connecting with support groups and mental health professionals, you can gain valuable insights, tools, and support to help both your loved one and yourself through this difficult time. Remember, seeking help is a sign of strength, not weakness, and taking this step can make a significant difference in your loved one's journey towards healing and recovery.

Advocating for the Well-Being of Your Loved One and Yourself

Advocating for the well-being of your loved one and yourself is crucial when supporting someone with chronic suicidal thoughts. It is important to remember that you cannot pour from an empty cup, so taking care of yourself is just as important as caring for your loved one.

One way to advocate for their well-being is to educate yourself on mental health and suicide prevention. This will help you better understand what your loved one is going through and how you can best support them. Attend workshops, read books, and speak with mental health professionals to gain a deeper understanding of their struggles.

Additionally, advocating for your loved one may involve seeking out resources and support systems that can help them in their journey towards healing. This could include therapy, support groups, crisis hotlines, and other mental health services. Encourage your loved one to seek help and offer to accompany them to appointments if needed.

It is also important to set boundaries and take care of your own mental health. Remember that you cannot save someone who does not want to be saved, and it is not your responsibility to fix them. Practice self-care, seek support from friends and family, and consider speaking with a therapist yourself to process your own emotions surrounding the situation.

Overall, advocating for the well-being of your loved one and yourself involves being proactive, seeking out resources, and taking care of your own mental health. Remember that you are not alone in this journey, and there are people and resources available to support you both.

| 10 |

Supporting a Loved One with Chronic Suicidal Thoughts

Long-Term Strategies for Supporting Your Loved One

In the midst of supporting a loved one with chronic suicidal thoughts, it is crucial to implement long-term strategies that promote stability, safety, and healing. These strategies are essential in providing ongoing support and guidance to your loved one as they navigate their journey towards recovery and wellness.

One key long-term strategy is to establish open and honest communication with your loved one.

Encourage them to express their thoughts and feelings without judgment, and actively listen to their concerns. By creating a safe space for dialogue, you can help your loved one feel heard and understood, which can ultimately strengthen your relationship and foster trust.

Another important long-term strategy is to educate yourself about mental health and suicide prevention. Take the time to learn about warning signs, risk factors, and available resources in order to better support your loved one. By equipping yourself with knowledge, you can more effectively advocate for your loved one's needs and connect them with appropriate professional help.

Additionally, it is essential to prioritize self-care and seek support for yourself as a concerned loved one. Taking care of your own well-being is crucial in maintaining your own mental and emotional health, which in turn enables you to provide better support to your loved one. Consider seeking therapy, joining a support group, or engaging in activities that bring you joy and relaxation.

By implementing these long-term strategies, you can effectively support your loved one with chronic suicidal thoughts and help them on their journey towards healing and recovery. Remember that you are not alone in this process, and reaching out for help is a sign of strength, not weakness. Together, we can create a supportive and caring environment for our loved ones as they navigate through their struggles with suicidal thoughts.

Managing Your Own Emotions and Mental Health

As a concerned loved one supporting someone with chronic suicidal thoughts, it is crucial to prioritize your own mental health and emotional well-being. It can be incredibly challenging and emotionally draining to support someone who is struggling with suicidal thoughts, so it is important to take care of yourself in order to effectively help your loved one. Here are some tips for managing your own emotions and mental health during this difficult time:

1. Seek support for yourself: It is essential to have a support system in place to lean on during this challenging time. Reach out to friends, family members, or a therapist for support and guidance. Talking to someone about your own feelings and fears can help you process your emotions and prevent burnout.
2. Set boundaries: While it is important to support your loved one, it is also crucial to set boundaries to protect your own mental health. It is okay to take breaks and prioritize your own needs, even if it means stepping back temporarily from the situation.
3. Practice self-care: Engage in activities that bring you joy and relaxation, such as exercise, meditation, or spending time in nature. Taking care of your physical and emotional well-being is essential for maintaining your own mental health.
4. Educate yourself: Learn about mental health and suicide prevention to better understand what your loved one is going through. Knowledge is power, and understanding the warning signs and risk factors

of suicide can help you provide better support.

5. Seek professional help if needed: If you are struggling to cope with your own emotions or feel overwhelmed by the situation, do not hesitate to seek help from a therapist or counselor. Your mental health is just as important as your loved one's, and it is okay to ask for help.

Remember, you cannot pour from an empty cup. Taking care of yourself is not selfish, but necessary in order to effectively support your loved one through their struggles with chronic suicidal thoughts. By managing your own emotions and mental health, you can be a stronger and more compassionate source of support for your loved one.

Finding Hope and Resilience in the Face of Chronic Suicidal Thoughts

Finding hope and resilience in the face of chronic suicidal thoughts can be a daunting task, but it is possible with the right support and resources. If you have a loved one who is struggling with chronic suicidal thoughts, it is important for you to understand that you are not alone in this journey. There are ways to help your loved one navigate through their struggles and find hope in the midst of their pain.

One of the most important things you can do for your loved one is to listen to them without judgment. Let them express their feelings and thoughts without trying to fix or change them. Sometimes, all a person needs is someone to listen and validate their emotions.

Encourage your loved one to seek professional help. Therapy and medication can be effective in treating chronic suicidal thoughts. Be there to support them in finding the right resources and treatment options.

Help your loved one build a support system. Encourage them to connect with friends, family, or support groups who can provide a listening ear and offer encouragement during difficult times.

Remind your loved one that there is hope for a brighter future. Encourage them to focus on the positive aspects of their life and to set small, achievable goals to work towards.

Above all, remember to take care of yourself as well. Supporting a loved one with chronic suicidal thoughts can be emotionally draining, so make sure to prioritize your own well-being and seek support for yourself when needed.

By finding hope and resilience in the face of chronic suicidal thoughts, you can help your loved one navigate through their struggles and work towards a brighter future together.

| 11 |

Helping a Loved One Through a Suicide Attempt and Recovery Process

Understanding the Aftermath of a Suicide Attempt

Understanding the aftermath of a suicide attempt is crucial for concerned loved ones who are supporting a person with chronic suicidal thoughts. It is a challenging and emotional time for both the individual who attempted suicide and their loved ones. It is important to approach this situation with empathy, understanding, and patience.

After a suicide attempt, the individual may experience a range of emotions such as guilt, shame, fear, and sadness. They may also feel overwhelmed by the consequences of their actions and may struggle to cope with the aftermath. As a concerned loved one, it is important to provide a supportive and non-judgmental environment for the individual to express their feelings and thoughts.

It is also important to encourage the individual to seek professional help and support. This may include therapy, counseling, medication, or other forms of treatment. It is crucial to work with mental health professionals to develop a safety plan to prevent future suicide attempts and to address any underlying issues that may have contributed to the attempt.

As a concerned loved one, it is important to take care of yourself as well. Supporting someone through a suicide attempt can be emotionally draining and overwhelming. It is important to seek support from friends, family, or a therapist to process your own emotions and experiences.

Remember, recovery from a suicide attempt is a journey that takes time and patience. By providing love, support, and understanding, you can help your loved one navigate through this difficult time and work towards healing and hope.

Providing Ongoing Support and Care During Recovery

Providing ongoing support and care during recovery is crucial when helping a loved one navigate through chronic suicidal thoughts. It is important to understand that recovery is not a linear process and setbacks may occur along the way. As a concerned loved one, your role is to provide unwavering support and understanding throughout this journey.

One of the most important aspects of providing ongoing support is to actively listen to your loved one without judgment. Allow them to express their feelings and thoughts without trying to fix them. Simply being present and offering a listening ear can make a significant difference in their recovery process.

Additionally, encourage your loved one to continue seeking professional help, whether it be through therapy, support groups, or medication management. Offer to accompany them to appointments or provide reminders for medication if needed. It is important for your loved one to have a strong support system in place to help them through the tough moments.

In times of crisis, it is important to have a safety plan in place. Work with your loved one to create a plan that outlines steps to take in case of a suicidal crisis. Include emergency contacts, coping strategies, and ways to access help during a crisis. Review and update this plan regularly to ensure it remains effective.

Lastly, take care of yourself as well. Supporting a loved one through chronic suicidal thoughts can be emotionally taxing. Make sure to prioritize self-care and seek support from friends, family, or a therapist if needed. Remember, you are not alone in this journey, and there are resources available to help both you and your loved one through this difficult time.

Promoting Healing and Growth After a Suicide Crisis

After experiencing a suicide crisis with a loved one, it is crucial to focus on promoting healing and growth in the aftermath. This period can be a challenging time for both the individual who attempted suicide and their support system. As concerned loved ones, it is important to provide a safe and nurturing environment for the individual to heal and recover.

One of the first steps in promoting healing and growth is to encourage open communication. It is essential for the individual to feel comfortable discussing their feelings and thoughts without fear of judgment or criticism. Listening actively and offering empathy can help the individual feel heard and understood.

Seeking professional help is also vital in

promoting healing and growth after a suicide crisis. Therapists, counselors, and support groups can provide the necessary tools and resources for the individual to work through their emotions and develop coping strategies. Encouraging the individual to attend therapy sessions regularly and participate in treatment plans can aid in their recovery process.

Creating a supportive and nurturing environment at home is another way to promote healing and growth. Encourage healthy habits such as exercise, proper nutrition, and sufficient sleep. Engage in activities together that bring joy and relaxation, such as going for walks, cooking meals together, or practicing mindfulness exercises.

It is important to be patient and understanding during this time of healing and growth. Recovery from a suicide crisis is a gradual process, and setbacks may occur. Encourage the individual to take things one day at a time and celebrate small victories along the way.

Remember, promoting healing and growth

after a suicide crisis requires ongoing support and understanding from concerned loved ones. By creating a safe and nurturing environment, encouraging open communication, seeking professional help, and fostering healthy habits, individuals can begin to heal and grow after experiencing a suicide crisis.

| 12 |

Enduring Hope in the Face of Suicidal Thoughts

Reflecting on Your Journey of Supporting a Loved One

As a concerned loved one, supporting someone who is struggling with chronic suicidal thoughts can be an emotional and challenging journey. It is important to take the time to reflect on your own experiences and emotions throughout this process in order to better understand and care for yourself as well as your loved one.

Reflect on how you have grown and changed throughout this journey. Have you developed new coping mechanisms or learned how to set boundaries to protect your own mental health? Recognize the strength and resilience that you have shown in supporting your loved one through their darkest moments.

Consider the impact that supporting a loved one with chronic suicidal thoughts has had on your relationships with others. Have you been able to lean on friends or family members for support, or has this experience caused strain in your other relationships? Reflect on how you can strengthen your support system and communicate your needs to those around you.

Take the time to acknowledge your own feelings of guilt, anger, frustration, and sadness. It is normal to experience a range of emotions when supporting someone through such a difficult time. Allow yourself to feel these emotions without judgment and seek out professional help or support groups if needed.

Remember to practice self-care and prioritize your own well-being. You cannot pour from an empty cup, so make sure to take time for yourself and engage in activities that bring you joy and relaxation.

By reflecting on your journey of supporting a loved one with chronic suicidal thoughts, you can gain a deeper understanding of your own needs and experiences. This self-awareness will not only benefit you but also enable you to continue providing the best possible support for your loved one.

Embracing Hope and Resilience in the Face of Adversity

In the face of adversity, it can be challenging to maintain hope and resilience, especially when supporting a loved one with chronic suicidal thoughts. However, it is crucial to embrace these qualities in order to effectively help your loved one through their struggles.

Hope is a powerful force that can provide light in the darkest of times. By holding onto hope, you can remind your loved one that there is a future worth fighting for, even when they may not see it themselves. Encouraging them to focus on the positive aspects of their life, no matter how small, can help them see that there is still reason to keep going.

Resilience is equally important when supporting a loved one with chronic suicidal thoughts. It is essential to be strong in the face of adversity and to remain steadfast in your support, even when things get tough. Remember that your loved one is going through a difficult time, and it is normal to feel overwhelmed at times. By practicing self-care and seeking support for yourself, you can better be there for your loved one when they need you most.

Together, hope and resilience can be powerful tools in helping your loved one through their struggles with suicidal thoughts. By embracing these qualities and staying committed to supporting your loved one, you can make a positive difference in their life and help them find the strength to keep going. Stay strong, stay hopeful, and never give up on your loved one.

Continuing to Advocate for Mental Health Awareness and Support

As concerned loved ones, it is crucial to continue advocating for mental health awareness and support for our loved ones who are struggling with chronic suicidal thoughts. The journey to recovery is not easy, and our support and advocacy play a significant role in their healing process.

One way to advocate for mental health awareness is by educating ourselves and others about the importance of seeking help for mental health issues. By raising awareness about the prevalence of mental health conditions and the effective treatments available, we can break the stigma surrounding mental illness and encourage our loved ones to seek the help they need.

Additionally, we can support mental health organizations and initiatives that provide resources and support for individuals struggling with suicidal thoughts. By volunteering our time, donating to these organizations, or participating in fundraising events, we can help ensure that those in need have access to the necessary support and resources.

It is also important to continue having open and honest conversations about mental health with our loved ones. By listening to their feelings and experiences without judgment, we can create a safe space for them to express themselves and seek help when needed.

Remember, advocating for mental health awareness and support is a continuous effort. By staying informed, supporting mental health initiatives, and fostering open communication with our loved ones, we can make a positive impact in their healing journey and contribute to a society that prioritizes mental health and well-being.

Final Note

Note: This book is intended for concerned loved ones who want to support their family members, friends, partners, parents, children, siblings, and coworkers through chronic suicidal thoughts and crises. It provides practical guidance, resources, and strategies for navigating the complex emotions and challenges that come with supporting someone struggling with suicidal ideation.

If you have a loved one who is experiencing chronic suicidal thoughts, it can be a difficult and overwhelming experience. You may feel helpless, scared, and unsure of how to best support them during this challenging time. This book is designed to provide you with the tools and knowledge you need to help your loved one through their struggles and to navigate the ups and downs that come with supporting someone dealing with suicidal ideation.

Throughout the pages of this book, you will find practical advice on how to communicate effectively with your loved one, how to create a safety plan, and how to access professional help when needed. You will also learn about the warning signs of suicide, how to recognize when your loved one is in crisis, and how to provide them with the support and care they need to stay safe.

Whether you are a parent, sibling, spouse, friend, or coworker, this book will provide you with the resources and strategies you need to support your loved one through their struggles with chronic suicidal thoughts. By arming yourself with knowledge and compassion, you can be a source of enduring hope for your loved one as they navigate this difficult journey.

RESOURCE INFORMATION

This QR Code is a listing of international resources for mental health crisis and more. Use your mobile device to scan it for up-to-date information.

www.ingramcontent.com/pod-product-compliance
Lightning Source LLC
Chambersburg PA
CBHW021332160726
47994CB00007B/2662

* 9 7 9 8 8 6 9 2 7 3 0 6 2 *